BIBLE VERSES

BELOVED WORDS FROM SCRIPTURE AND INSPIRATIONAL PHOTOGRAPHS

AN INTERACTIVE BOOK FOR MEMORY-IMPAIRED ADULTS

Shadowbox Press books are designed to facilitate a rewarding reading experience by providing entertainment, education, and comfort to individuals diagnosed with Alzheimer's disease, Parkinson's disease, stroke, brain injury, or other memory-impairment condition.

For more information, go to www.shadowboxpress.com

Shadowbox Press, established in 2009, is an independent publisher committed to providing high-quality, interactive books to the memory-impaired adult audience.

Published by Shadowbox Press, LLC
P.O. Box 268
Richfield, OH 44286
www.shadowboxpress.com

Chief Creative Director: Matthew Schneider
Product Development Director: Deborah Drapac, BSN, RN

This book is intended to be informational and should not be considered a substitute for advice from a health care professional. The authors and the publisher expressly disclaim responsibility for any adverse effects arising from the use or application of the information contained in this book.

Publisher's Cataloging-in-Publication data

Schneider, Matthew John.
    Bible verses : beloved words from scripture and inspirational photographs, an interactive book for memory-impaired adults / Matthew Schneider ; Deborah Drapac, BSN, RN.
    p. cm.
    ISBN-13: 978-0-9831577-1-7; ISBN-10: 0-9831577-1-5
1. Alzheimer's disease—Patients—Rehabilitation. 2. Dementia—Patients—Rehabilitation.
3. Caregivers. 4. Self-care, Health. I. Drapac, Deborah Ann. I. Title.

RC523.S37 2011
362.196'831—dc22   2010917058

Manufactured in China

Bible Verses

Beloved Words from Scripture and Inspirational Photographs

An Interactive Book for Memory-Impaired Adults

Matthew Schneider
Deborah Drapac, BSN, RN

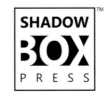

Shadowbox Press, LLC
Richfield, Ohio

INTRODUCTION

Shadowbox Press began with one simple mission: to develop interactive products for memory-impaired adults to revisit and share memories through the reading experience.

Storytelling is a valuable form of communication that connects one another and allows us to relate to each other on a personal level. It sparks the imagination, promotes self-reflection, and provides a way to find meaning in our experiences.

We have published a collection of books that offer a variety of subject matter designed to engage the user with meaningful content and provide a connection to both the past and present. Every effort has been made in the development of these books to maximize the experience for the user. They may be read independently or shared with an individual by a caregiver, loved one, staff member, or volunteer.

Our books offer a rewarding reading experience that stimulates the mind and offers engagement opportunities for the user. You will find inspiring words, inviting photographs, innovative conversation prompts, and unique activities to facilitate an interactive, multi-sensory experience. These books can generate meaningful communication and provide the feeling of well-being associated with sharing experiences and stories together. Through engagement, you may discover common backgrounds and interests, realize mutual bonds, and/or participate in a quality conversation.

We believe the reading experience should be shared at all stages of life, and sincerely hope that our passion for books touches your heart. We trust that you will find meaning, delight, and comfort in sharing a title from our collection of Shadowbox Press books. May you explore and discover memories, share experiences, and reflect on the value and purpose of life.

At Shadowbox Press, we welcome feedback from our readers and listeners. Please contact us at www.shadowboxpress.com to share your reading experiences, stories, and suggestions for future books.

ABOUT THIS BOOK

This book has been created to provide an interactive reading experience for a memory-impaired adult. It is designed to encourage socialization, evoke memories, prompt conversation, and supply mental and physical stimulation, thereby improving the overall quality of life for the individual user.

There are a variety of benefits from using this book. By encouraging engagement through personal reminiscing; a feeling of empowerment, an elevated mood, a positive self-image, and/or a reduced level of depression may result. In addition, a caregiver's presence, support, and attention can communicate acceptance, reassurance, and affection to a memory-impaired adult.

This book is comprised of three sections:

1. The STORY is the foundation of the book and is designed to entertain, inform, inspire, and/or educate. It features inviting photographs paired with engaging, large-print text written in clear, concise, and easy-to-read sentences. The content is intended to cultivate an interest in reading, evoke memories, and encourage opportunities to reminisce.

2. CONVERSATION STARTERS are questions that directly correlate to an individual set of pages from the STORY. Each series of inquiry-based questions are designed to prompt a dialog from experiences, events, and/or relationships. Engaging in conversation provides a memory-impaired adult the opportunity to share special memories and unique experiences from their life.

3. ACTIVITIES are exercises based on sensory stimulation, creative expression, and physical movement. These simple but purposeful activities correspond to the overall theme of the book, and are designed to provide additional mental and physical enrichment. Participation in a variety of activities is essential to overall good health and emotional well-being.

This book does not have to be read in its entirety to provide a benefit. Each set of pages is intended to encourage thinking, stimulate emotions, and evoke unique memories. An individual page may trigger a response and lead to a meaningful conversation. Through the reading and reminiscing process, the user can share his or her unique life story, express personal values, and, perhaps, reveal a legacy to pass on to future generations.

INTERACTION GUIDELINES

Communication is what connects us to each other. Because memory impairment slowly diminishes communication skills, it creates distinct challenges in how an individual communicates their thoughts and emotions, as well as comprehend what is being communicated to them. The key to managing the behaviors associated with memory impairment lies in the methods of engagement by caregivers and others. It is important to adapt our thinking and behaviors to create a more comfortable environment for a memory-impaired adult.

Guidelines for a successful reading experience:

- Locate a quiet, comfortable setting, free of distractions, for the reading experience.
- Before beginning, take a moment and allow yourself to relax. Imagine a connection between the voice and the story and reflect upon the importance of the time spent together.
- Always approach the individual from the front and make eye contact.
- Position your head at the same level as the individual's head. Bend your knees or sit down to reach a correct level.
- Smile whenever it's appropriate. A connection can grow from a smile.
- Present the book to the individual and invite them to share in the reading experience.
- Read aloud slowly, in an adult tone with a clear, calm, inviting, and enthusiastic voice, pausing after each sentence.
- Speak in short, direct sentences, focusing on a single idea at a time.
- Focus on central words and ideas, emphasizing the ones that may evoke memories.
- Point out key aspects of the photographs and invite the individual to share their thoughts.
- Include your own comments and encourage the individual to share their memories by prompting them with the CONVERSATION STARTERS.
- Ask only one question at a time, allowing the individual to answer it before continuing.
- Be aware of nonverbal cues. It is often possible to recognize a connection by observing facial expressions and/or body language.
- After a response, either verbal or nonverbal, acknowledge the contribution with positive reinforcement and encourage further discussion.
- Remember to be patient, as it may take longer for a memory-impaired adult to fully process and respond to a particular word, phrase, idea, or image.
- At times, engagement may become challenging. However, always treat the individual with dignity and respect.

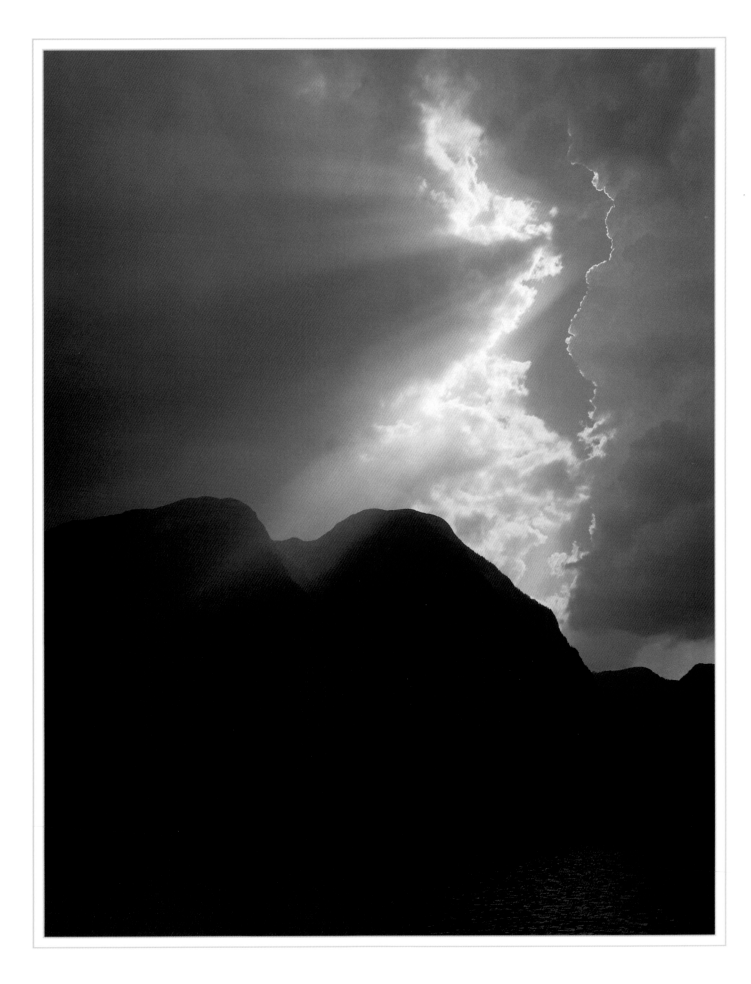

IN THE BEGINNING GOD CREATED
THE HEAVENS AND THE EARTH.

—GENESIS 1:1

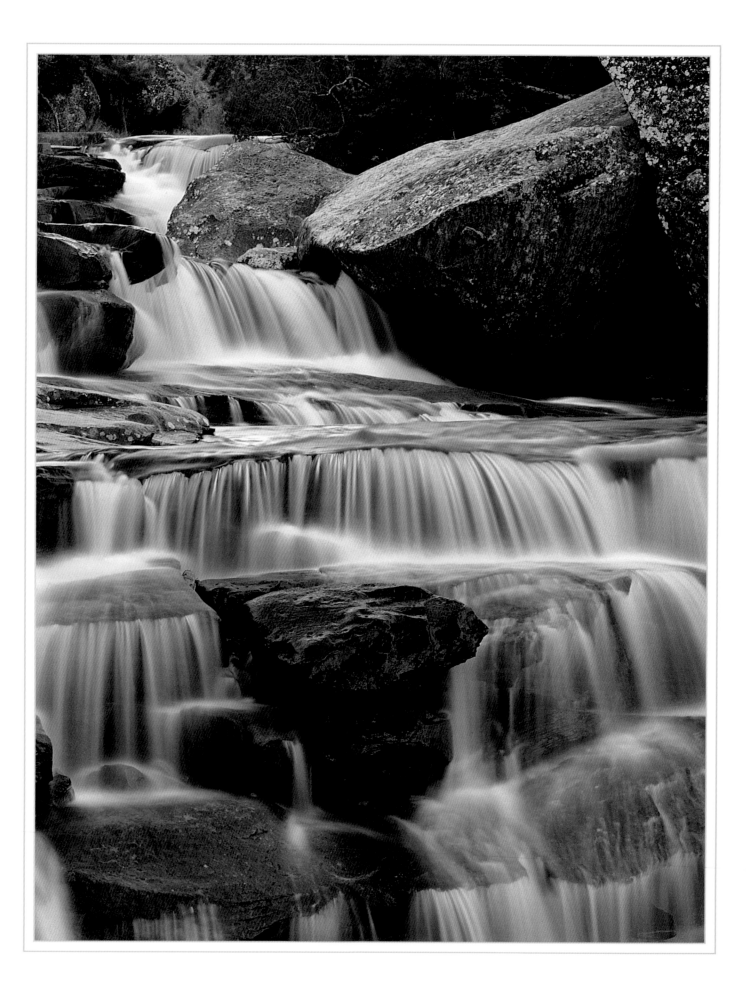

Jesus answered, "Most assuredly, I say to you, unless one is born of water and the Spirit, he cannot enter the kingdom of God.

—John 3:5

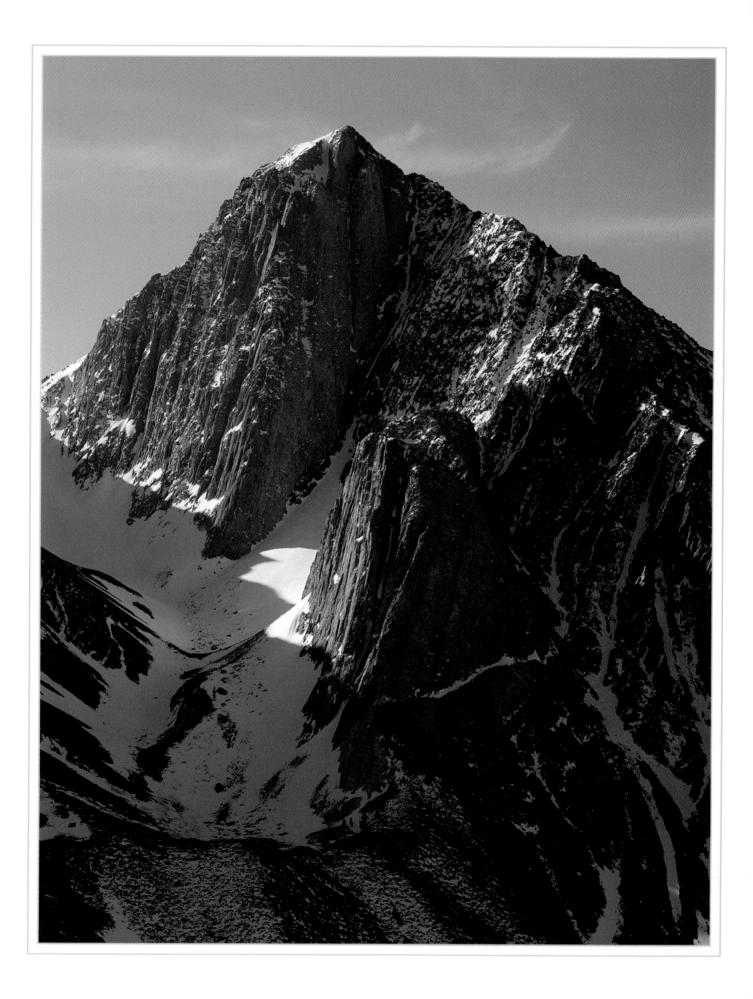

I CAN DO ALL THINGS THROUGH CHRIST
WHO STRENGTHENS ME.

—PHILIPPIANS 4:13

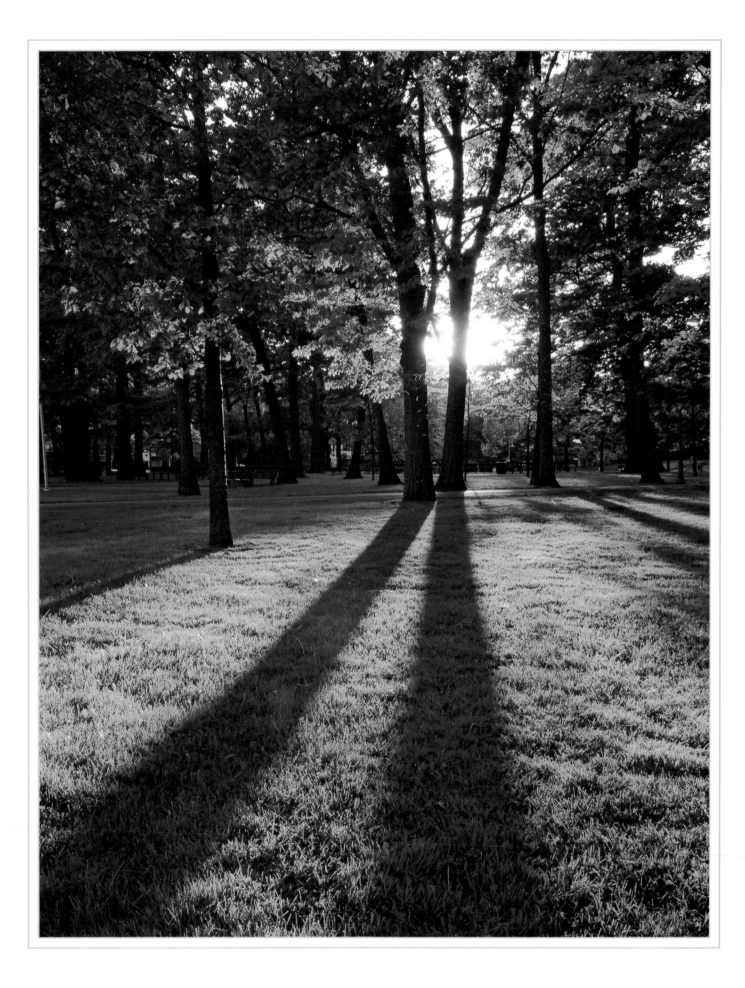

LET THE FIELD BE JOYFUL, AND ALL
THAT IS IN IT. THEN ALL THE TREES
OF THE WOODS WILL REJOICE
BEFORE THE LORD.
FOR HE IS COMING, FOR HE IS COMING
TO JUDGE THE EARTH.
HE SHALL JUDGE THE WORLD
WITH RIGHTEOUSNESS,
AND THE PEOPLES WITH HIS TRUTH.

—PSALM 96:12–13

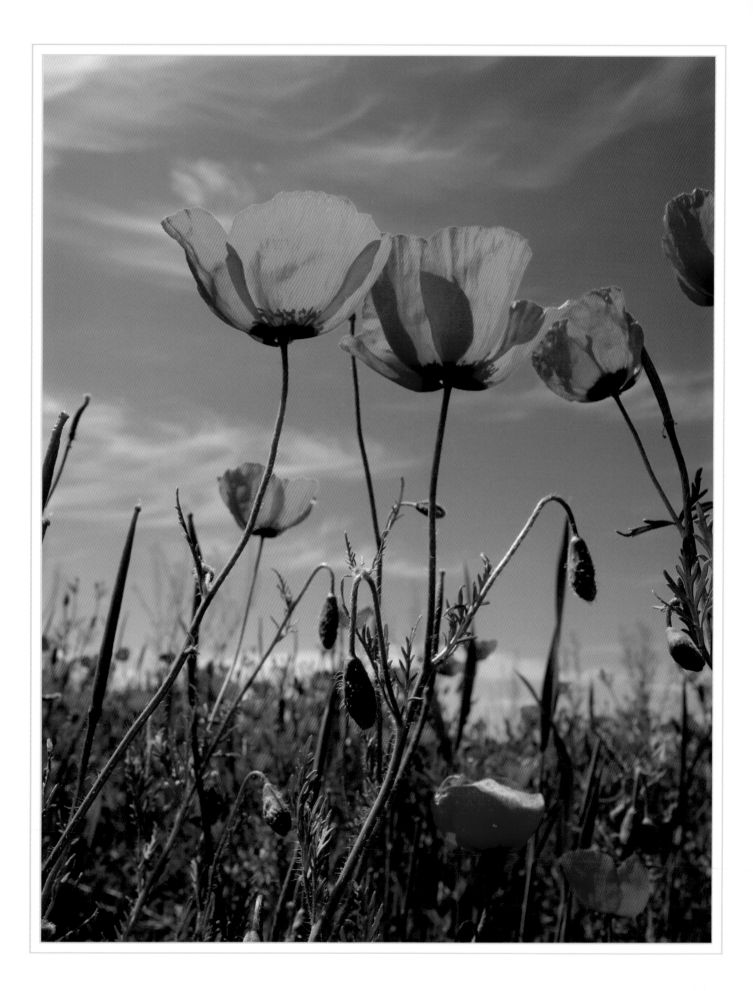

But the fruit of the Spirit is love, joy, peace, longsuffering, kindness, goodness, faithfulness, gentleness, self-control. Against such there is no law.

—Galatians 5:22–23

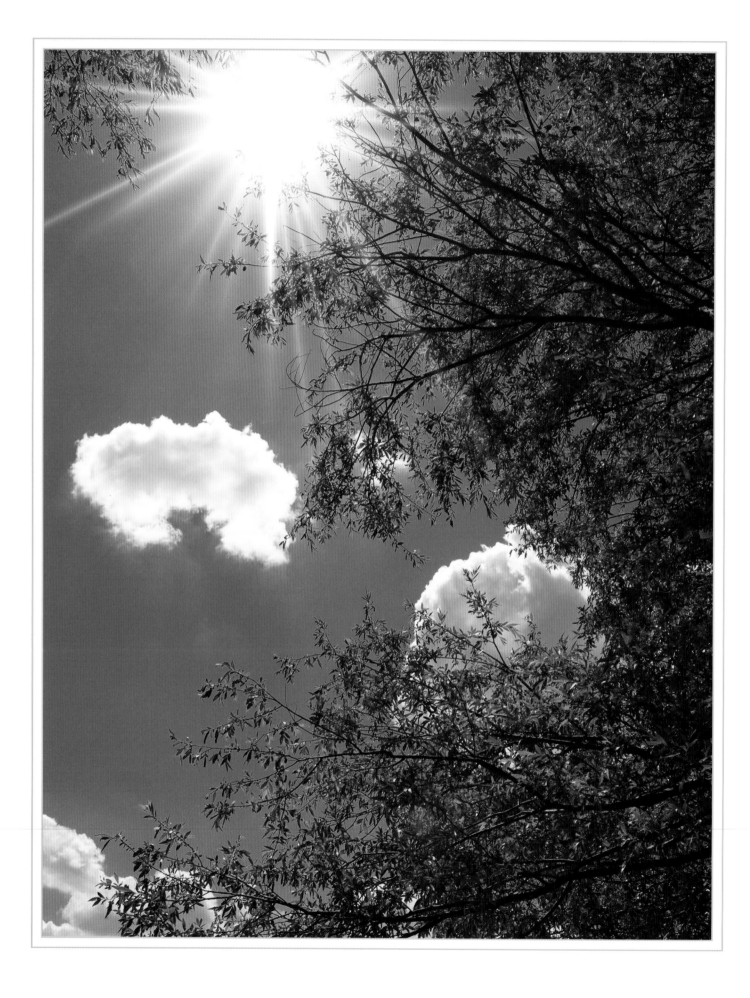

For God so loved the world
that He gave His only begotten Son,
that whoever believes in Him
should not perish
but have everlasting life.

—John 3:16

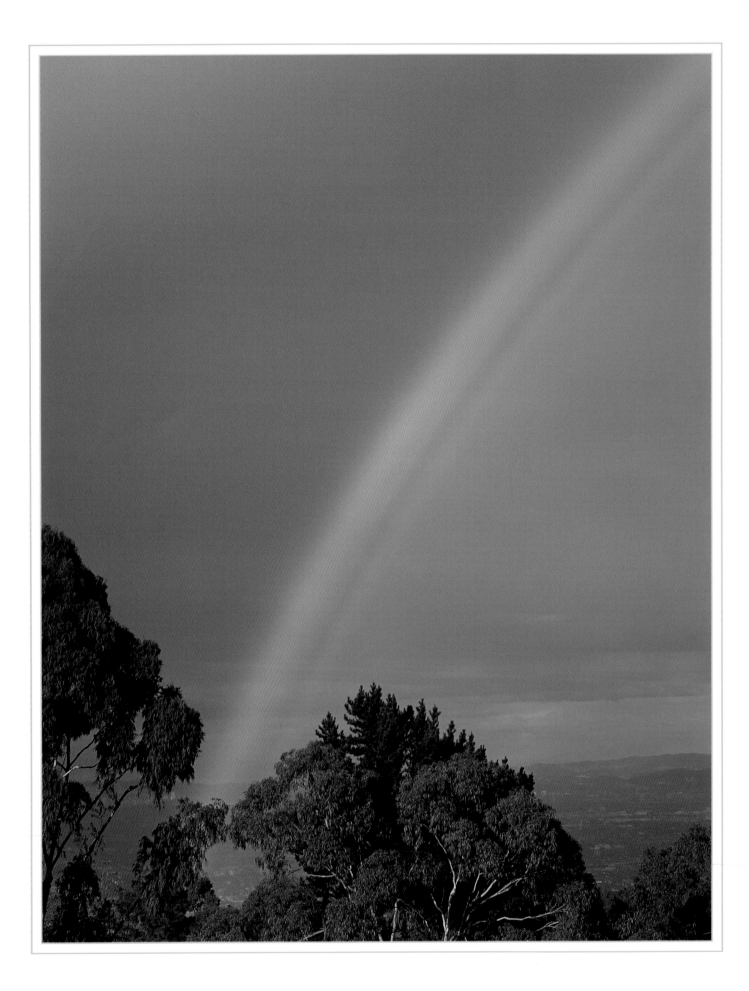

THE RAINBOW SHALL BE IN THE CLOUD,
AND I WILL LOOK ON IT TO REMEMBER
THE EVERLASTING COVENANT BETWEEN
GOD AND EVERY LIVING CREATURE
OF ALL FLESH THAT IS ON THE EARTH."

—GENESIS 9:16

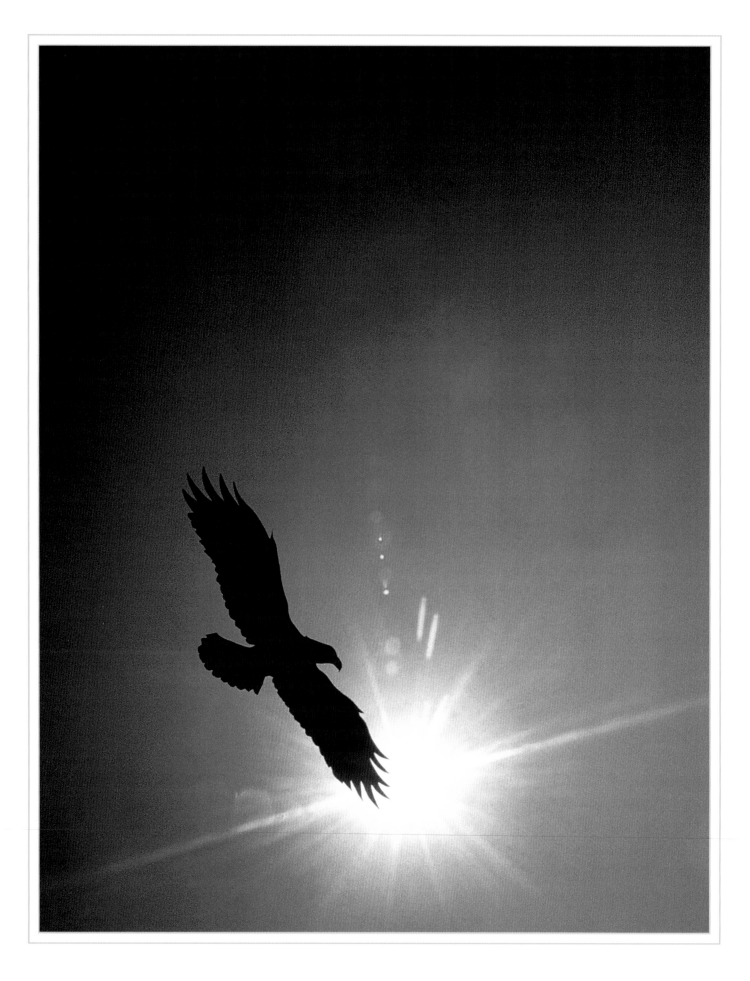

But seek first the kingdom of God and His righteousness, and all these things shall be added to you.

—Matthew 6:33

From the rising of the sun
to its going down
The LORD's name is to be praised.

—Psalm 113:3

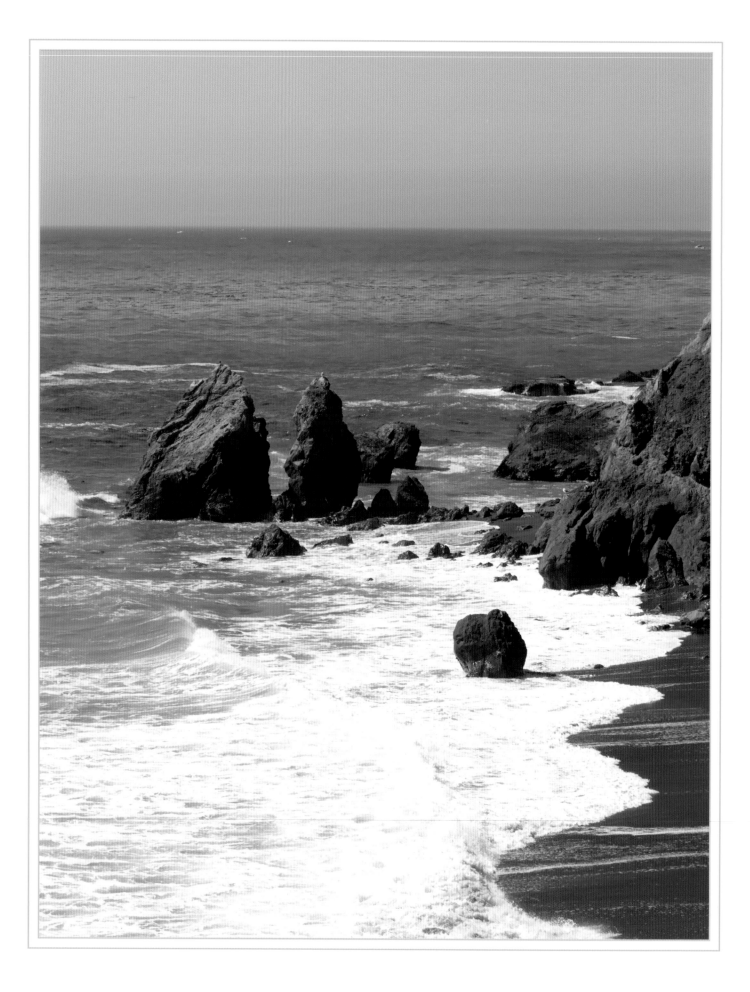

Go therefore and make disciples
of all the nations, baptizing them
in the name of the Father
and of the Son
and of the Holy Spirit,

—Matthew 28:19

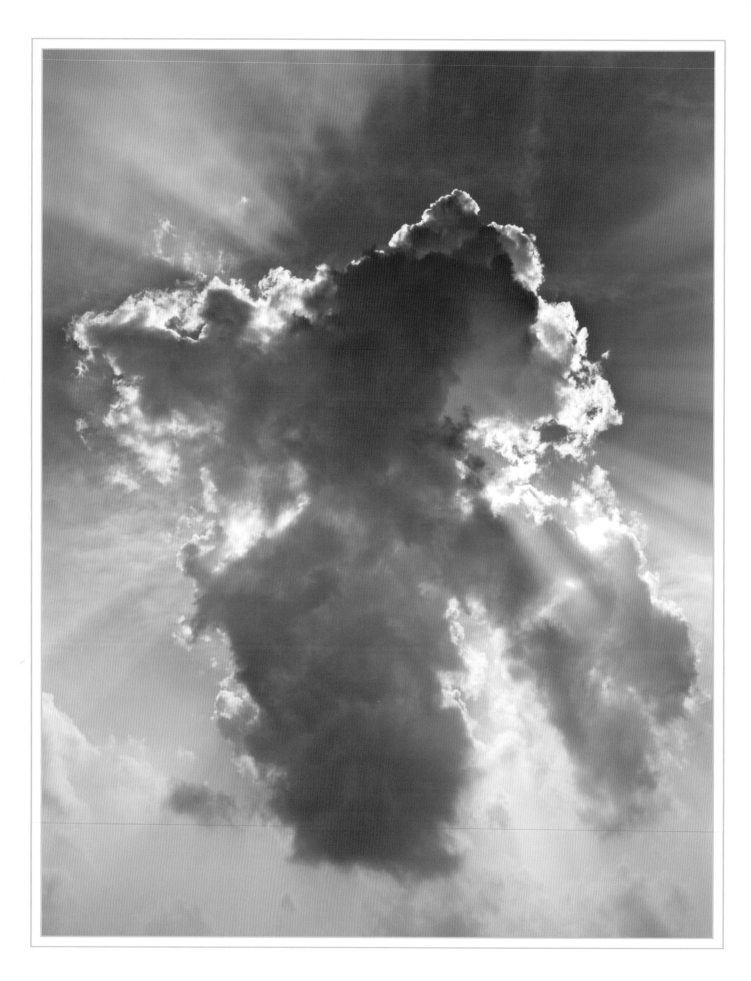

Now faith is the substance
of things hoped for, the evidence
of things not seen.

—Hebrews 11:1

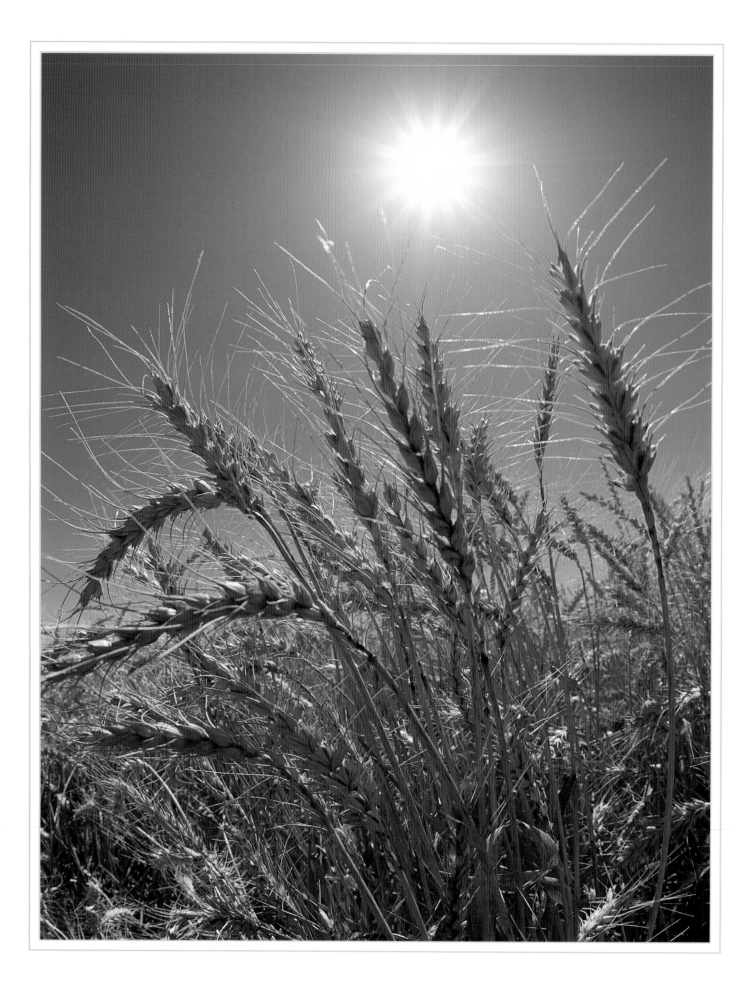

And let us not grow weary
while doing good, for in due season
we shall reap if we do not lose heart.

—Galatians 6:9

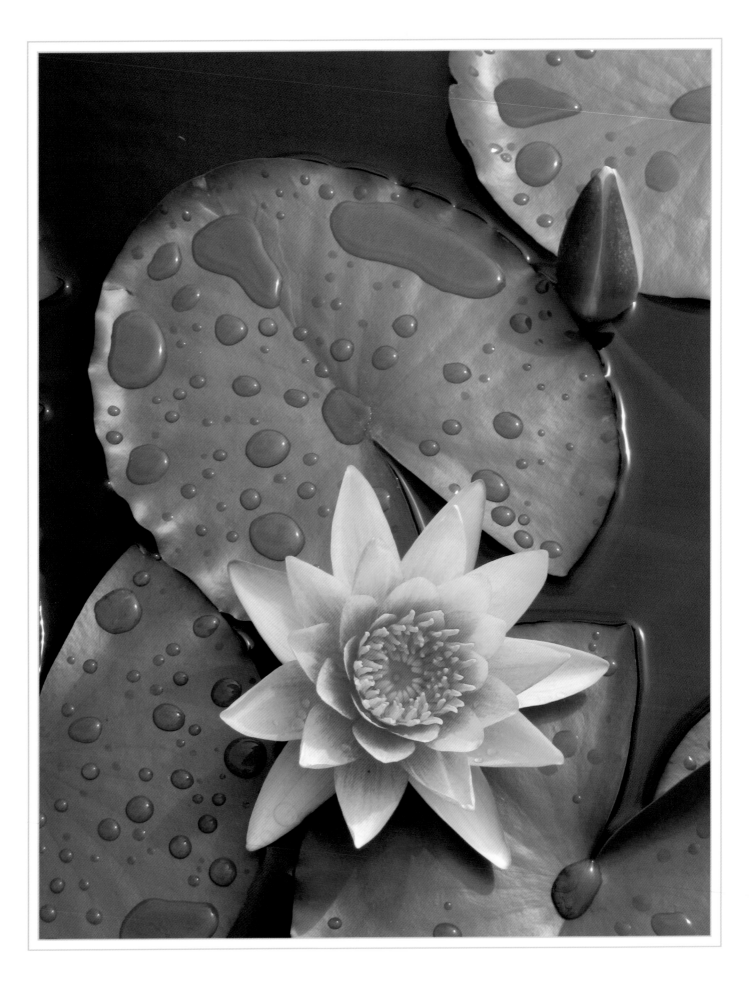

AND WE KNOW THAT ALL THINGS
WORK TOGETHER FOR GOOD
TO THOSE WHO LOVE GOD,
TO THOSE WHO ARE THE CALLED
ACCORDING TO HIS PURPOSE.

—ROMANS 8:28

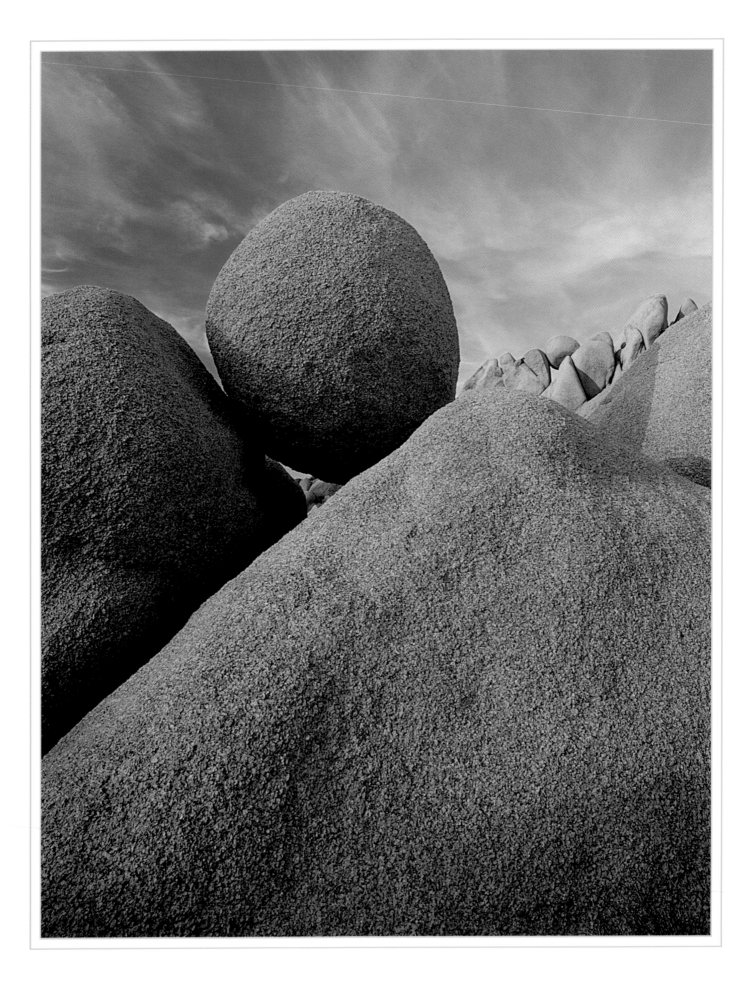

THE LORD IS MY ROCK AND MY FORTRESS
AND MY DELIVERER; MY GOD, MY STRENGTH,
IN WHOM I WILL TRUST; MY SHIELD
AND THE HORN OF MY SALVATION,
MY STRONGHOLD.

—PSALM 18:2

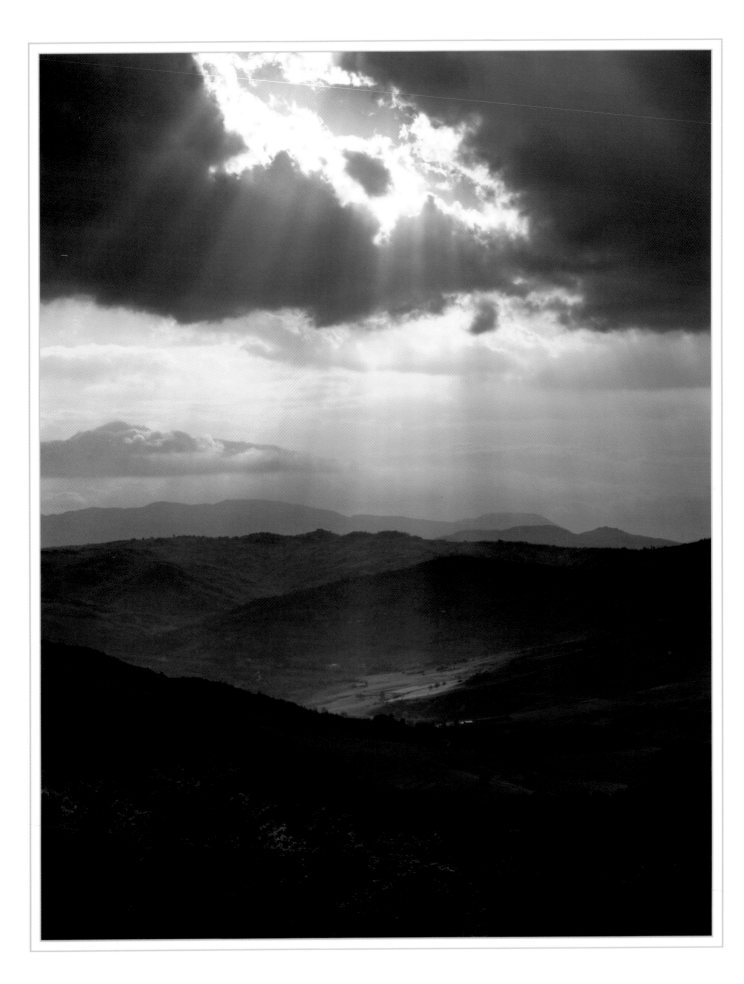

THAT IF YOU CONFESS WITH YOUR
MOUTH THE LORD JESUS AND BELIEVE
IN YOUR HEART THAT GOD
HAS RAISED HIM FROM THE DEAD,
YOU WILL BE SAVED.

—ROMANS 10:9

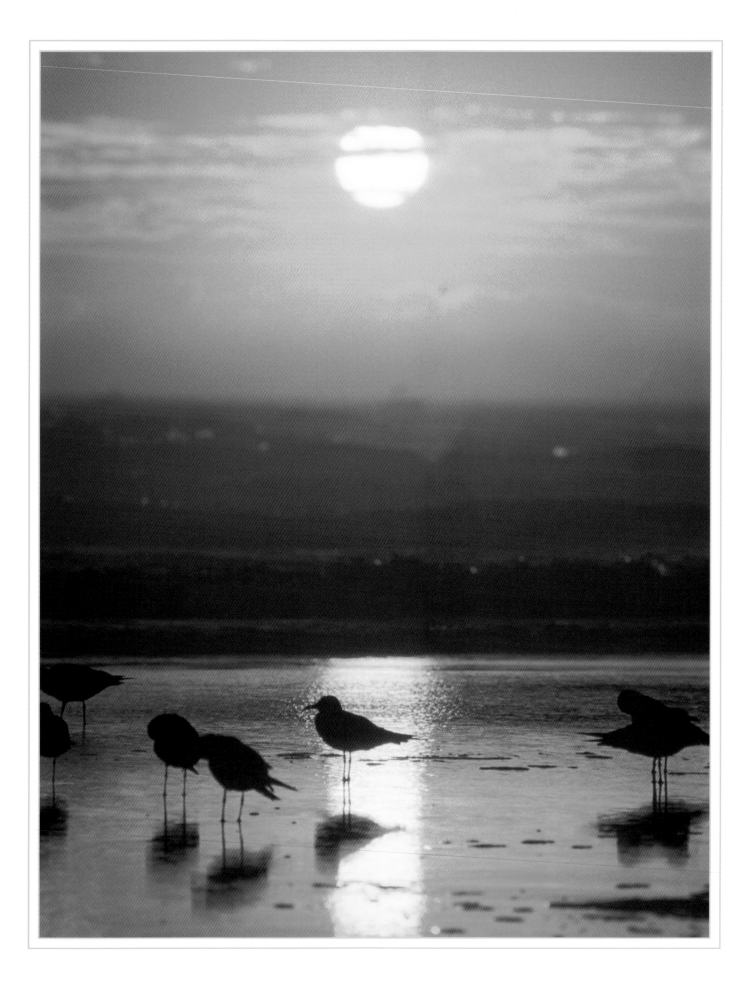

FOR BY GRACE YOU HAVE BEEN SAVED
THROUGH FAITH, AND THAT NOT OF
YOURSELVES; IT IS THE GIFT OF GOD,

—EPHESIANS 2:8

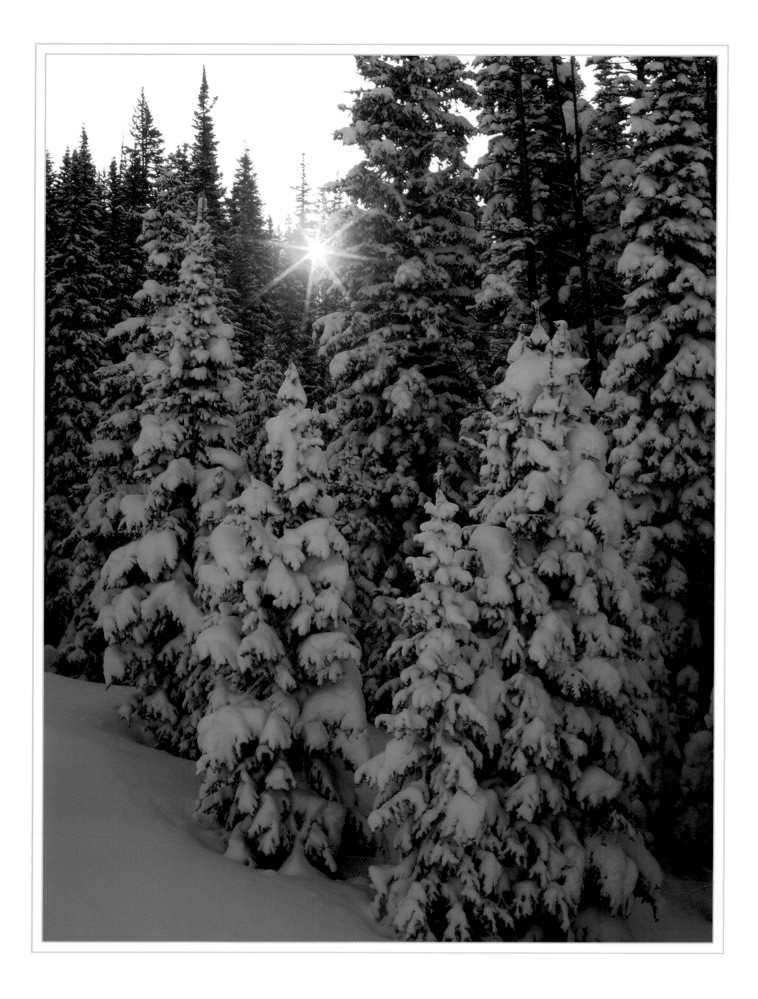

FOR THERE IS BORN TO YOU THIS DAY
IN THE CITY OF DAVID A SAVIOR,
WHO IS CHRIST THE LORD.

—LUKE 2:11

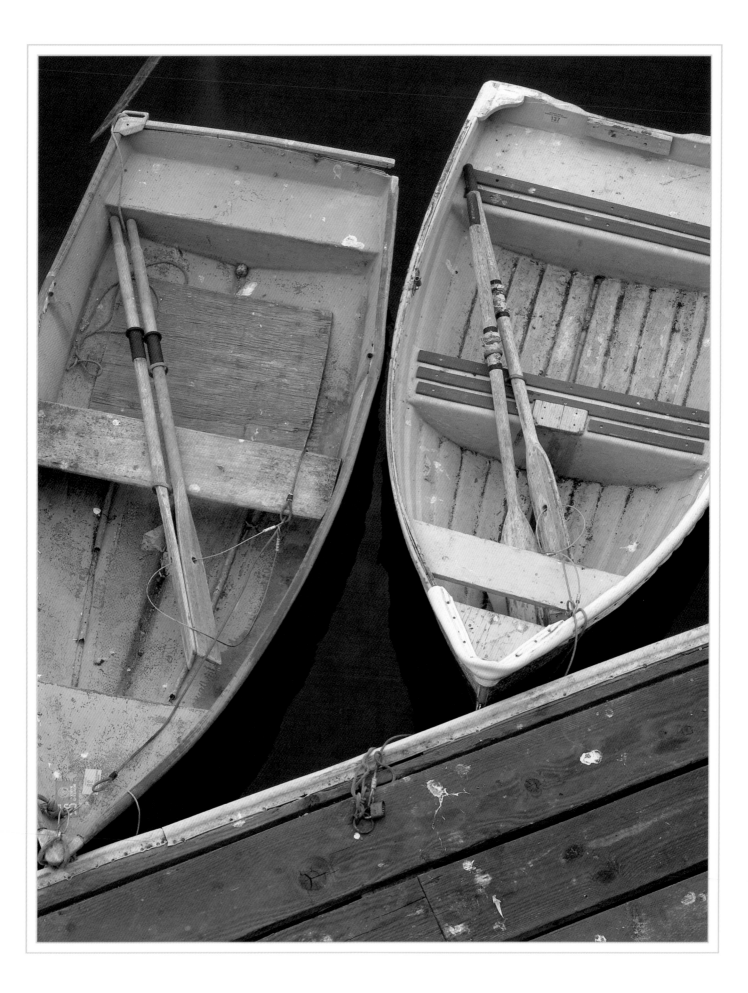

COME TO ME, ALL YOU WHO
LABOR AND ARE HEAVY LADEN,
AND I WILL GIVE YOU REST.

—MATTHEW 11:28

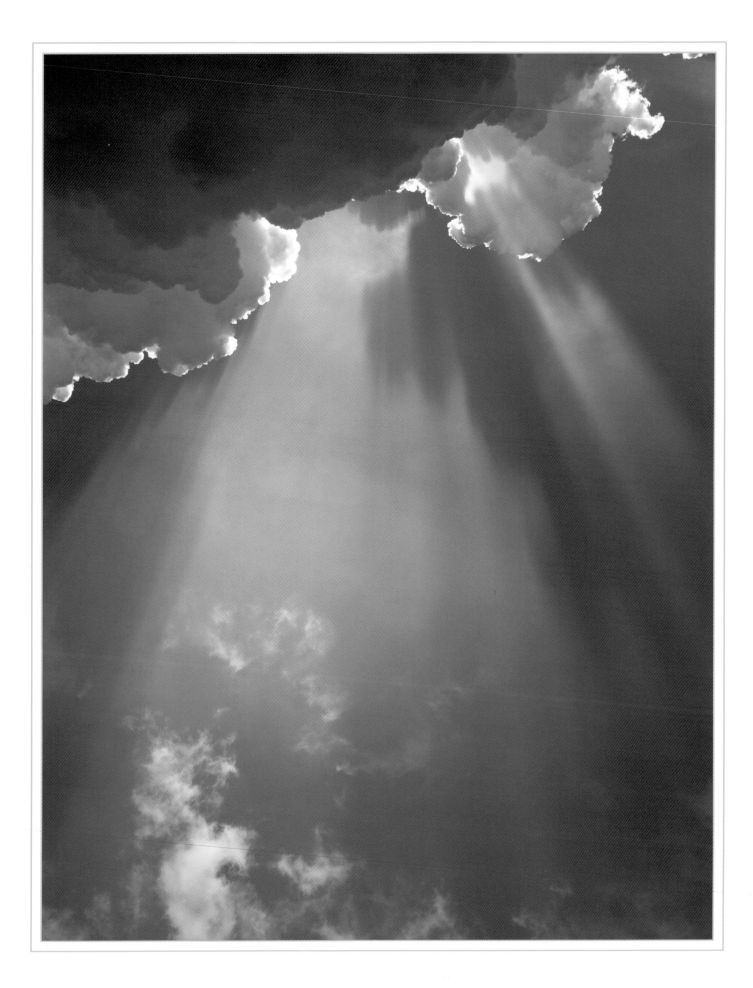

YOUR MERCY, O LORD,
IS IN THE HEAVENS;
YOUR FAITHFULNESS
REACHES TO THE CLOUDS.

—PSALM 36:5

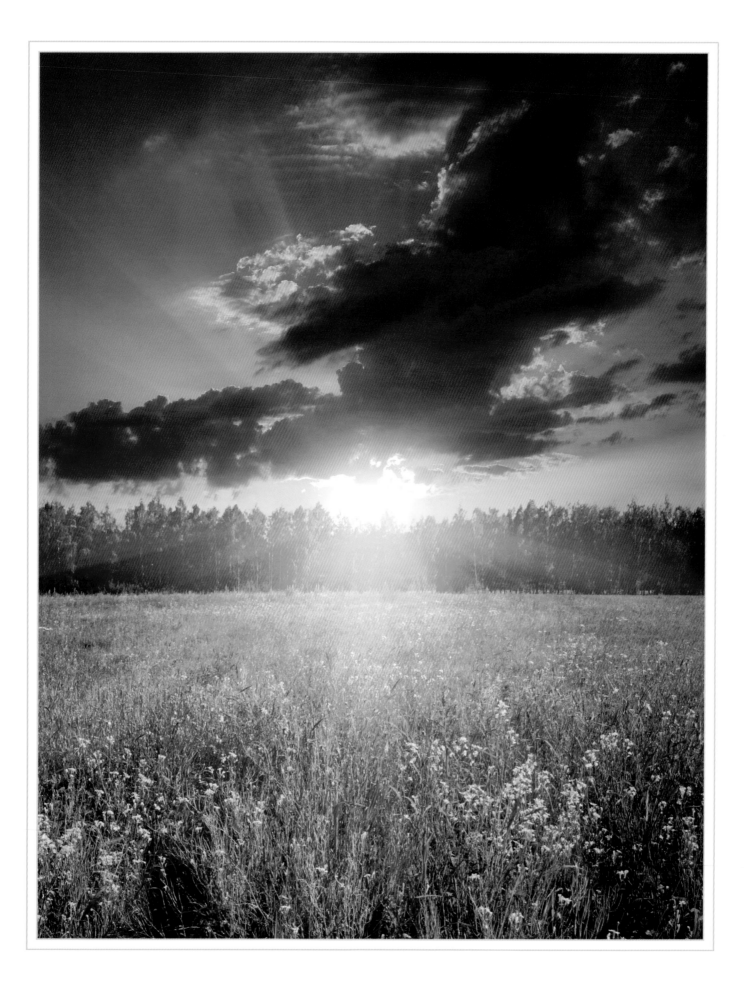

Trust in the LORD
with all your heart,
And lean not
on your own understanding;
In all your ways
acknowledge Him,
And He shall direct your paths.

—Proverbs 3:5–6

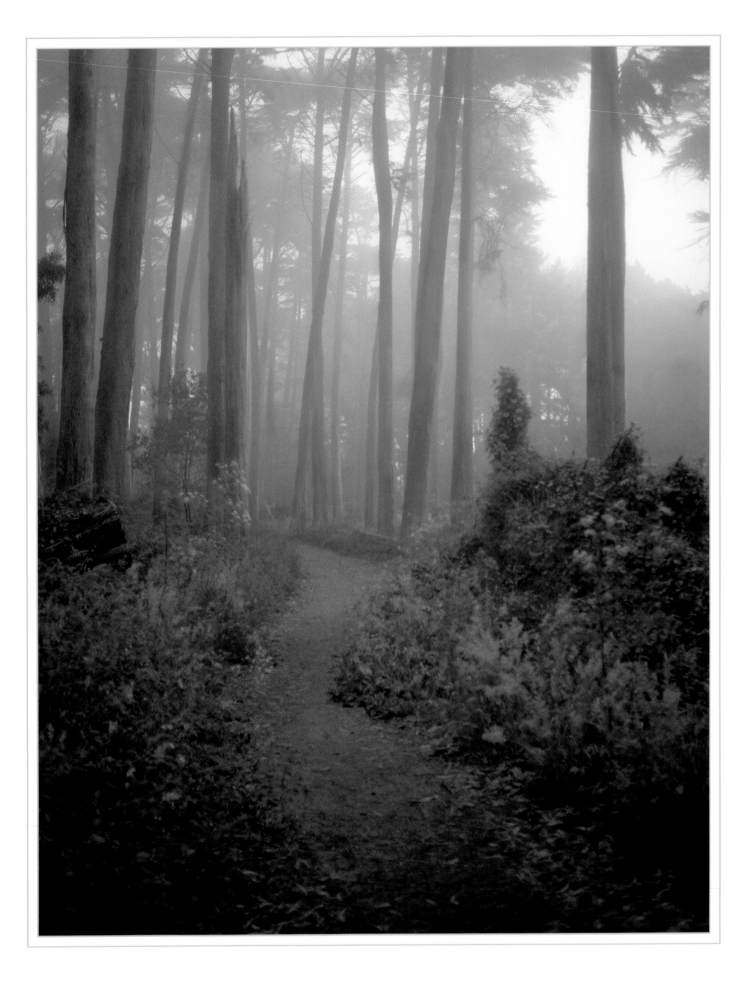

Jesus said to him, "I am the way, the truth, and the life. No one comes to the Father except through Me.

—John 14:6

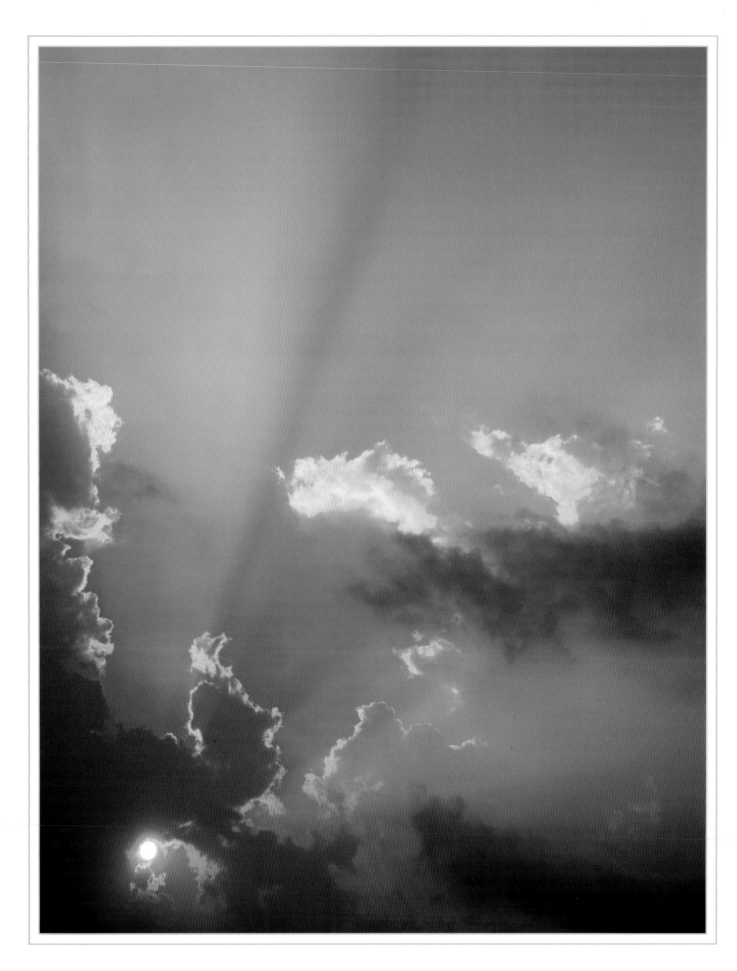

Let your light so shine before men, that they may see your good works and glorify your Father in heaven.

—Matthew 5:16

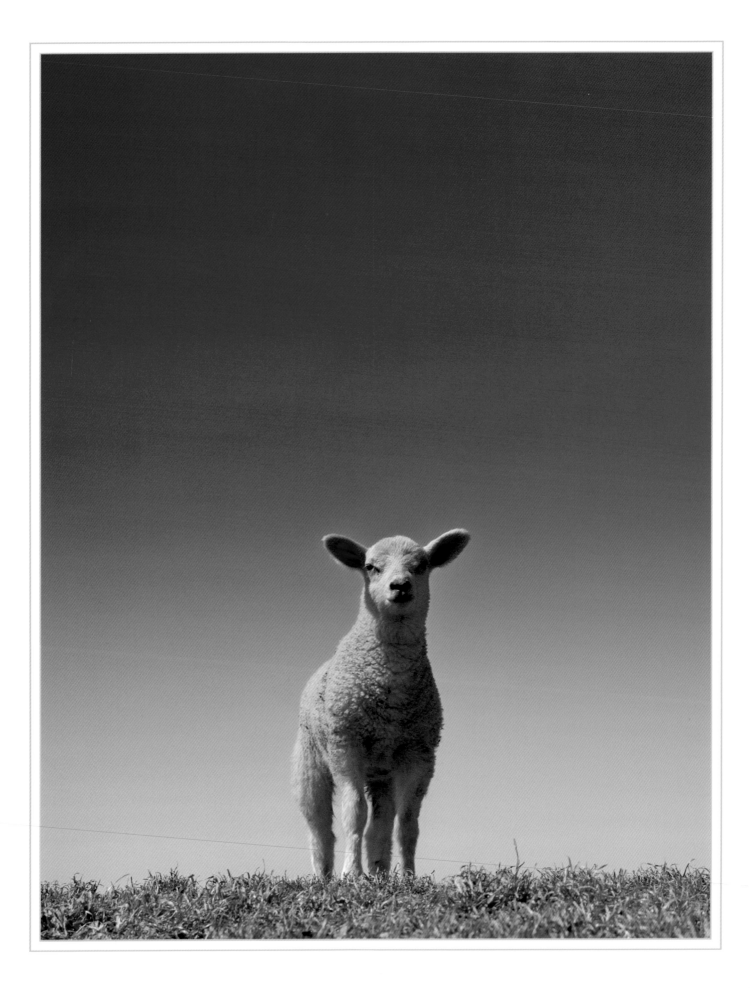

THE LORD IS MY SHEPHERD;
I SHALL NOT WANT.
HE MAKES ME TO LIE DOWN
IN GREEN PASTURES;
HE LEADS ME BESIDE THE STILL WATERS.
HE RESTORES MY SOUL;
HE LEADS ME IN THE PATHS
OF RIGHTEOUSNESS
FOR HIS NAME'S SAKE.

—PSALM 23:1–3

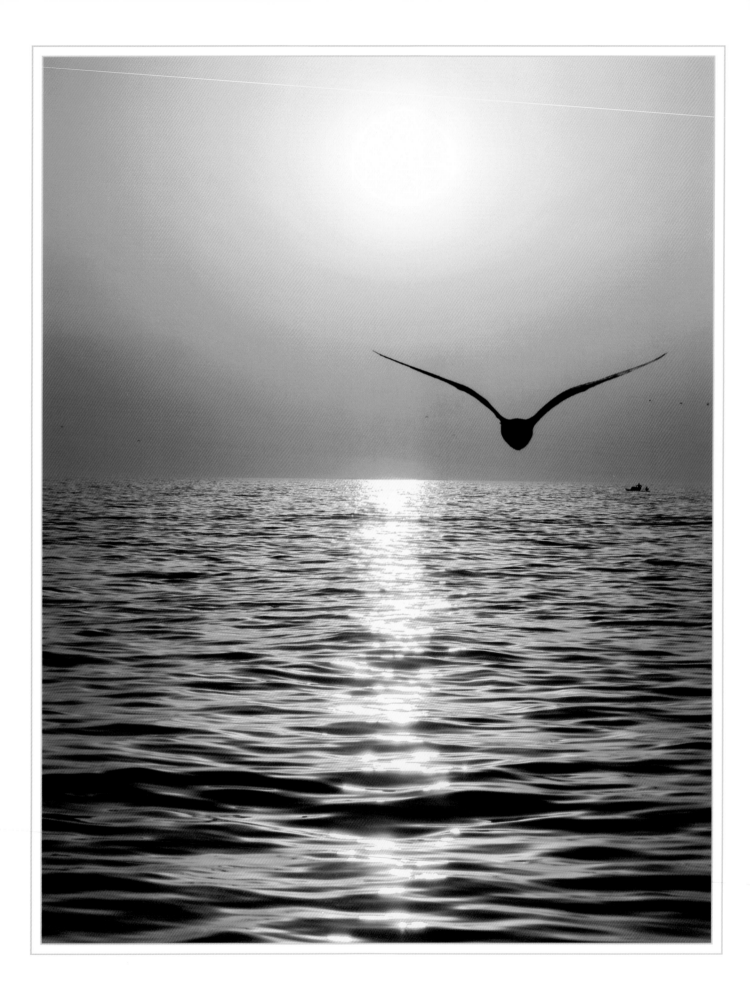

The grace of our Lord Jesus Christ be with you all. Amen.

—Revelation 22:21

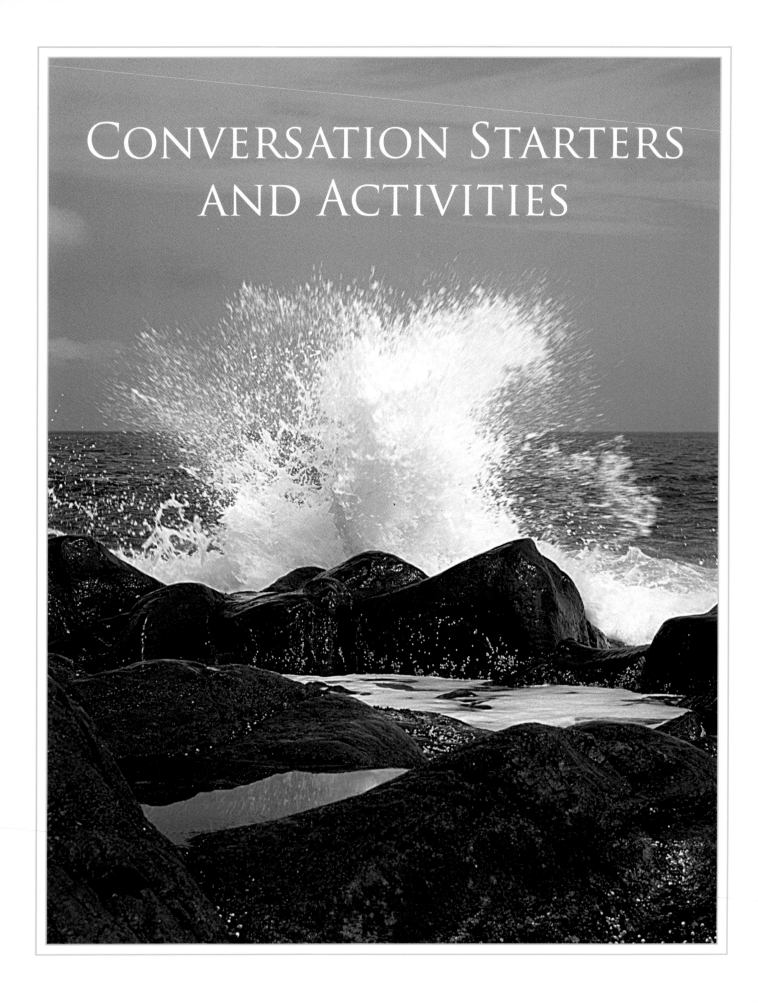

CONVERSATION STARTERS AND ACTIVITIES

CONVERSATION STARTERS are designed to engage the user and encourage self-expression. They consist of a combination of close-ended (yes or no) and open-ended questions. Each series of four questions correlate to an individual set of pages and are intended to be referenced during the reading experience. Each question is designed to prompt a response by the user from a photograph, word, phrase, or idea from the STORY. After a response from a specific question, either verbal or nonverbal, encourage further discussion on that particular subject. Urging the user to elaborate on an experience allows them to connect to the story and to the caregiver.

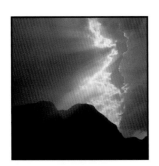

Did you know that the Bible is the best-selling book of all time?

Do you like to read the Bible?

Did you have a family Bible?

What part of God's creation of the world do you find the most magnificent?

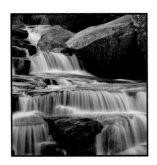

Did you know that Jesus was baptized in the Jordan River?

Have you been baptized?

Did you go to church with your family when you were a child?

Where did you learn about God?

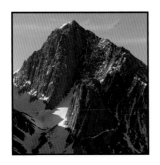

Did you know that Moses received the Ten Commandments on Mount Sinai?

Did you memorize the Ten Commandments as a child?

Did you pray when you were growing up?

What religious movies have you watched?

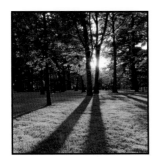

Did you know that the longest book of the Bible is the Book of Psalms?

Do you talk to God about your deepest feelings?

Do you like to sing hymns?

How did you get to church?

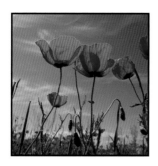

Did you know that the Book of Galatians is a letter from the apostle Paul to the early Christians?

Did you get married in a church?

Have you ever belonged to a Bible study group?

What did you wear to church on Sundays?

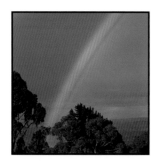

Did you know that John 3:16 is the most well-known verse in the New Testament?

Did you have a cross on the wall of your childhood home?

Do you believe that Jesus died on the cross for us?

Where did your family attend Good Friday services?

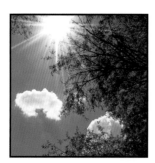

Did you know that Noah knew the flood had ended when a dove returned with an olive leaf?

Do you like rainbows?

Did you have a book of Bible stories?

What Bible stories did you enjoy as a child?

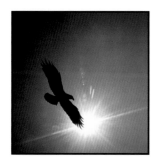

Did you know that the Book of Matthew is the first book of the New Testament?

Did you obey your parents when you were growing up?

Do you believe that God answers prayers?

Who taught you right from wrong when you were a child?

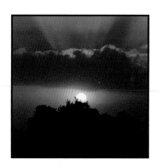

Did you know that the Book of Psalms is a collection of prayers and songs?

Do you like to watch sunrises and sunsets?

Have you ever attended an Easter sunrise service?

What did your family do to prepare for Easter?

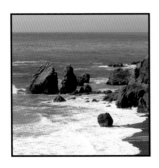

Did you know that Jesus was baptized by his cousin, John the Baptist?

Was water used in your church for blessings?

Did you ever attend a church service with relatives when you were growing up?

What prayers do you recite daily?

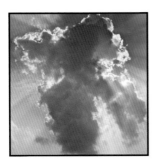

Did you know that the Bible was written by over 40 different authors?

Did you have a prayer book when you were a child?

Do you believe that God watches over you?

What religious occasions or events did you celebrate at church?

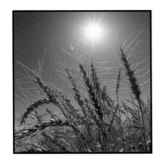

Did you know that Jesus turned two loaves of bread and two fish into a meal that fed 5,000 people?

Did you say grace before meals when you were growing up?

Have you ever attended a dinner at your church?

What church festivals have you attended?

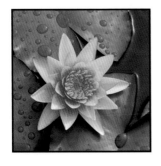

Did you know that the water lily was used to decorate Solomon's temple?

Did your family pray together?

Did you memorize prayers and Bible verses when you were growing up?

What time of day do you prefer to pray?

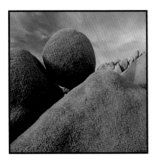

Did you know that the name Peter comes from the Greek word meaning "rock"?

Have you ever sung in a church choir?

Did your church have a bulletin every Sunday?

What musical instruments were used during your church services?

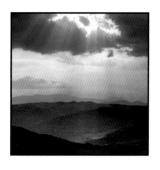

Did you know that the Book of Romans was written by the apostle Paul?

Did you go to church on Easter Sunday with your family when you were growing up?

Was your church decorated with lilies on Easter Sunday?

What Easter traditions did your family share together?

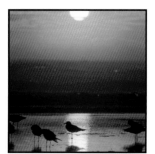

Did you know that the Bible mentions birds about 300 times?

Have you ever attended a church retreat?

Do you believe that God is forgiving?

Who inspired you to follow God?

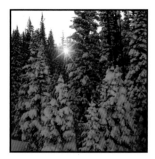

Did you know that Jesus, the son of Mary and Joseph, was born in a stable in the town of Bethlehem?

Have you ever been to a candlelight service?

Do you like to sing Christmas carols?

How did your family celebrate Christmas when you were growing up?

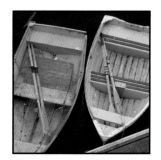

Did you know that Jesus chose four fishermen to be his apostles: Peter, Andrew, James, and John?

Did you say prayers before you went to sleep when you were a child?

Did you eat a special dinner on Sundays when you were growing up?

What did your family do on Sundays?

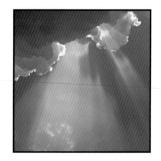

Did you know that Luke tells us that Jesus will be coming in a cloud when he returns to Earth?

Do you like gospel music?

Do you believe in Heaven?

What religious programs have you watched on television?

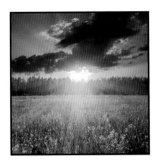

Did you know that the Book of Proverbs tells us that it is better to have wisdom than gold?

Did your parents teach you to trust in God?

Did you ask your parents questions about God when you were growing up?

Whom do you pray for in your family?

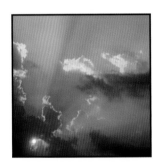

Did you know that Jesus taught others about God's love by preaching, storytelling, and performing miracles?

Has God given you special gifts or talents?

Did you ever pray for God's guidance when you had to make a difficult decision?

What was your life's work?

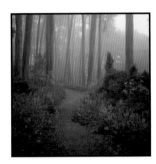

Did you know that the Gospel of Matthew is the most quoted book in the New Testament?

Do you like to see light shine through a stained glass window?

Did you or your family volunteer at church?

What did you pray for when you were a child?

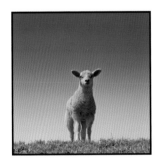

Did you know that Jesus calls himself the "Good Shepherd" in the New Testament?

Do the words of Jesus comfort you?

Has reading the Bible enriched your life?

What person in the Bible would you most like to meet?

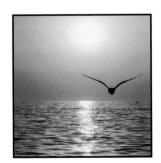

Did you know that the Book of Revelation is the last book of the Bible?

Do you believe God loves you?

Do you think it's important to teach children about God?

What are you grateful for in your life?

ACTIVITIES are designed to enrich the user's life by introducing diversity into the daily routine through mental and physical engagement. They are intended to be performed under the supervision of a caregiver. Caution should be exercised when outdoors, in unfamiliar surroundings, or when using potentially harmful materials and/or equipment. Selection of an appropriate activity is dependent on individual ability; however, the user may participate or benefit from observing another individual perform the activity.

SENSORY STIMULATION ACTIVITIES

Participate in a worship service. Attend a church service, watch a service on television, or listen to a religious program on the radio. Experience personal spiritual enrichment by giving glory and praise to God.

Bake bread. Locate a simple bread recipe. Measure and mix the ingredients, knead the dough, let it rise, place the dough in a bread pan, allow it to rise again, and bake. Pray the "Our Father" and give thanks for the food that nourishes the body and soul. Enjoy the aroma as the bread bakes, and experience the feeling of comfort that prayer provides.

Watch the sun rise. Sit outdoors and feel the warmth of the sun as it rises above the horizon. Reflect on the sights and sounds of nature and God's great love for the world.

Listen to Christian music. Select popular pieces from a variety of genres, including hymns, worship, gospel, instrumental, and contemporary. Sing, whistle, hum, clap, or tap feet to the music. Witness the hope, promise, and joy music brings to a spiritual life.

Display a lily for the Easter season. Purchase an Easter lily, place it in a prominent location, and enjoy its delicate beauty and fragrance. After the lily has finished blooming, plant the bulb outdoors and watch for it to sprout in the spring.

Visit an art museum. Explore American and European religious artwork. View a variety of paintings and sculptures, and identify Biblical and spiritual themes. Study the subject matter of each of the pieces. Reflect on the feelings of faith and devotion that they evoke.

Start a freshwater fish tank. Purchase freshwater fish and a small aquarium kit or goldfish and a fishbowl. Experience the relaxing and rewarding hobby of watching and caring for fish.

Make Christmas cookies. Cut sugar-cookie dough into holiday shapes with cookie cutters. Bake the cookies, remove them from the oven, and allow them to cool. Decorate the cookies with Christmas-colored frosting and sprinkles. Organize a cookie exchange with family and friends.

Create a prayer corner. Select a space in the living area and place a Bible, religious picture, cross, and/or other significant religious articles on a small table. Pray in this sacred space daily as an exercise in faith.

CREATIVE EXPRESSION ACTIVITIES

Create a prayer jar. Decorate a plastic jar with religious symbolism. Cut several strips of paper and write the name of a family member, friend, or neighbor on each one. Place them in the jar. Draw a name from the jar each day and pray for that person.

Decorate eggs for Easter. Purchase an egg-coloring kit. Hard-boil the eggs and use egg dyes and wax crayons to create decorative designs on the eggs. Refrigerate the eggs and enjoy them on their own, mix them into a salad, or make deviled eggs or egg salad.

Create a scrapbook photo album. Choose photographs of Christmas, Easter, baptisms, weddings, etc. Arrange the items on the pages and adhere them using a glue stick. Write a brief description below each photo. Put the finished pages in page protectors and place them in an album. Review the scrapbook and relive memories of church gatherings and family celebrations.

Design placemats for a dinner table. Use pens, markers, paints, or stencils and apply symbols of faith such as a cross, a fish, praying hands, etc. Include an inspirational verse from Scripture. Laminate the placemat and use at mealtimes as a reminder of God's bounty.

Make a prayer bracelet. String colored beads on beading thread and attach a jewelry clasp to each end. Hold or wear the bracelet and recite a traditional prayer, mantra, or Scripture passage while touching each successive bead. Experience the joy and security that prayer provides.

PHYSICAL MOVEMENT ACTIVITIES

Tour a historic church. Take a walking tour and examine the beauty of the church's historic architecture, stained glass windows, altar, tapestries, organ, pews, etc. Learn about the church's history and its heritage.

Create a bird garden. Plant purple coneflowers, zinnias, sunflowers, etc. to attract a variety of birds. Tend the garden and enjoy God's creatures as they visit the garden. Use this place of beauty for prayer and spiritual meditation.

Attend a church picnic, carnival, or festival. Experience the joyous atmosphere of a church-sponsored event. Sample the food, have a cold drink, feel the rhythm of the music, and enjoy spending time with family, friends, and members of the congregation.

Take a nature walk through a park or nature center in the spring. Look for spring wildflowers and signs of new growth on the plants and trees. Enjoy the spirituality of nature's sights and sounds.

Help clean a church. Volunteer to dust, polish, sweep, clean door handles, organize prayer books, etc. Experience the spiritual atmosphere of the church while working.